Sirtfood Diet Cookbook

Lunch Recipes

Delicious and Healthy Recipes for Anyone.

Get Lean by Activating Your Skinny Gene. Lose Weight and Feel Great

Melany Morris

2nd Edition

Table of Contents

Introduction

How It Works

The Diet Has Two Easy-To-Follow Phases:

Phase 1: This lasts for seven days. During the first three days, you should have three sirtfood green juices and one full meal rich in sirtfoods – a total of 1,000 calories. On days four to seven, you should increase your calorie intake to 1,500 by having two green juices and two meals daily.

Phase 2: This 14-day maintenance phase is intended to help you lose weight steadily. You can eat three balanced sirtfood-rich meals every day, plus one green juice.

Eating Plan

The Sirtfood diet has been formulated to last for three weeks, although the principles of the diet can be applied long-term to help with maintenance. How do you start the Sirtfood diet?

First Phase (Days 1–3):

❖ Limit calorie intake to 1,000 calories a day during the first three days of the diet
❖ Drink three glasses of sirtfood green juice each day
❖ Eat one sirtfood rich meal per day
❖ 15-20g dark chocolate(85% cocoa) is permitted

First Phase (Days 4–7):

❖ Limit calorie intake to 1,500 calories a day (500 more calories than during the first three days) on days 4–7
❖ Drink two sirtfood green juices per day
❖ Eat two sirtfood-rich meals per day
❖ 15-20g dark chocolate(85% cocoa) is permitted

Second Phase (Lasts Two Weeks):

There isn't a strict long-term plan once you finish the first week. You're encouraged to eat three balanced meals and to continue drinking sirtfood juice.

To maintain your results, it's recommended that you still include lots of sirtfoods in your diet, while sticking to mostly balanced, plant-based meals. This plan can be continued indefinitely, as long as you eat enough calories to support your needs.

What Are Some Examples Of Balanced Meals That Include Sirtfood-Rich Foods?

❖ Cooked buckwheat muesli with berries and walnuts
❖ Stir-fry made with whole grains, veggies, turmeric, and tofu
❖ Kale salad made with chicken and veggies like tomatoes and onions, dressed with olive oil and herbs
❖ Sirtfood snacks can include a bit of dark chocolate, dried fruits or berries, "energy bites," greek yogurt, or raw veggies dipped in hummus
❖ The two phases can be repeated whenever you like for a fat-loss boost.

What Happens After The Second Phase? And Is This Kind Of Diet Sustainable?

The idea of "certifying" meals are for those who have completed phase one and two but still want to continue on the Sirtfood path. It involves taking your favorite dish and giving it a Sirtfood twist. Recipes include everyday favorites such as chicken curry, chilli-con-Carne, pizza, and pancakes.

The Sirtfood Diet is not designed to be a one-off 'diet' but rather a way of life. You are encouraged, once you've completed the first 3 weeks, to continue eating a diet rich in Sirtfoods and to continue drinking your daily green juice. There are now many Sirtfood Diet recipe books available, with recipes for lots more Sirtfood-rich main meals, as well as recipes for alternatives to the green juice and more hints and tips for following the Sirtfood Diet. There are even some recipes for Sirtfood desserts! Phases 1 and 2 can be repeated as and when necessary for a health boost, or if things have gone a bit off track.

Getting Started

Daily juices are essential to the Sirtfood Diet. So make sure you have a juicer. You'll also need three key ingredients.

Matcha is a powdered green tea and an important ingredient in green juices. It's readily available online if your local health food shop doesn't stock it. Similarly, lovage – a herb in the green juice recipe – can sometimes seem hard to find. But it's easy to buy seeds online to grow it in a pot on a windowsill.

Finally, buckwheat. It's a fantastic alternative to more common grains, but most supermarkets mix buckwheat and wheat in their products. You're more likely to find 100 percent buckwheat products in your local health food store.

The Health Benefits

There is growing evidence that sirtuin activators may have a wide range of health benefits as well as building muscle and suppressing appetite. These include improving memory, helping the body better control blood sugar levels, and cleaning up the damage from free radical molecules that can accumulate in cells and lead to cancer and other diseases.

'Substantial observational evidence exists for the beneficial effects of the intake of food and drinks rich in sirtuin activators in decreasing risks of chronic disease,' said Professor Frank Hu, an expert in nutrition and epidemiology at Harvard University in a recent article in the journal Advances In Nutrition. A Sirt food diet is particularly suitable as an anti-aging regime.

Although sirtuin activators are found all through the plant kingdom, only certain fruits and vegetables have large enough amounts to counting as Sirt foods. Examples include green tea, cocoa powder, the Indian spice turmeric, kale, onions, and parsley. Many of the fruit and vegetables on display in supermarkets, such as tomatoes, avocados, bananas, lettuce, kiwis, carrots, and cucumber, are rather low in sirtuin activators. This doesn't mean that they aren't worth eating, though, as they provide lots of other benefits.

A remarkable finding of one Sirt food diet trial is that participants lost substantial weight without losing muscle. It was common for participants to gain muscle, leading to a more defined and toned look. That's the beauty of sirtfoods; they activate fat burning but also promote muscle growth, maintenance, and repair. This is in complete contrast to other diets where weight loss typically comes from both fat and muscle, with the loss of muscle slowing down metabolism and making weight regain more likely.

In terms of weight loss and boosting metabolism, people may have experienced a seven-pound weight loss on the scales, but in my experience, this will be fluid. Burning and losing fat takes time so it is extremely unlikely this weight loss is a loss of fat. I would be very cautious of any diet that recommends fast and sudden weight loss as this simply isn't achievable and will more than likely be a loss of fluid. As soon as people return to their regular eating habits, they will regain the weight. Slow and steady weight loss is the key and for this, we need to restrict calories and increase our activity levels. Eating balanced regular meals made up of low GI foods, lean protein, fruit, and vegetables, and keeping well hydrated is the safest way to lose weight.'

What Are These Magical 'Sirtfoods'? The Twenty Most Common Include:

❖ kale

❖ red wine

❖ strawberries

❖ onions

- ❖ soy

- ❖ parsley

- ❖ extra virgin olive oil

- ❖ dark chocolate (85% cocoa)

- ❖ matcha green tea

- ❖ buckwheat

- ❖ turmeric

- ❖ walnuts

- ❖ arugula (rocket)

- ❖ bird's eye chili

- ❖ lovage

- ❖ Medjool dates

- ❖ red chicory

- ❖ blueberries

- ❖ capers

- ❖ coffee

The diet is divided into two phases; the initial phase lasts one week and involves restricting calories to 1000kcal for three days, consuming three sirtfood green juices, and one meal rich in sirtfoods each day. The juices include kale, celery, rocket, parsley, green tea, and lemon. Meals include turkey escalope with sage, capers and parsley, chicken and kale curry, and prawn stir-fry with buckwheat noodles. From days four to seven, energy intakes are increased to 1500kcal comprising of two sirtfood green juices and two sirtfood-rich meals a day. Although the diet promotes healthy foods, it's restrictive in both your food choices and daily calories, especially during the initial stages. It also involves drinking juice, with the amounts suggested during phase one exceeding the current daily guidelines.

The second phase is known as the maintenance phase which lasts 14 days where steady weight loss occurs. The authors believe it's a sustainable and realistic way to lose weight. However, focusing on weight loss is not what the diet is all about – it's designed to be about eating the best foods nature has to offer. Long term they recommend eating three balanced sirtfood rich meals a day along with one sirtfood green juice.

Dietitian Emer Delaney Says:

'At first glance, this is not a diet I would advise for my clients. Aiming to have 1000kcal for three consecutive days is extremely difficult and I believe the majority of people would be unable to achieve it. Looking at the list of foods, you can see they are the sort of items that often appear on a 'healthy food list', however it would be better to encourage these as part of a healthy balanced diet. Having a glass of red wine or a small amount of chocolate occasionally won't do us any harm – I wouldn't recommend them daily. We should also be eating a mixture of different fruits and vegetables and not just those on the list.

'In terms of weight loss and boosting metabolism, people may have experienced a seven-pound weight loss on the scales, but in my experience, this will be fluid. Burning and losing fat takes time so it is extremely unlikely this weight loss is a loss of fat. I would be very cautious of any diet that recommends fast and sudden weight loss as this simply isn't achievable and will more than likely be a loss of fluid. As soon as people return to their regular eating habits, they will regain the weight. Slow and steady weight loss is the key and for this, we need to restrict calories and increase our activity levels. Eating balanced regular meals made up of low GI foods, lean protein, fruit, and vegetables, and keeping well hydrated is the safest way to lose weight.'

1. <u>Asparagus Mushroom Melt</u>

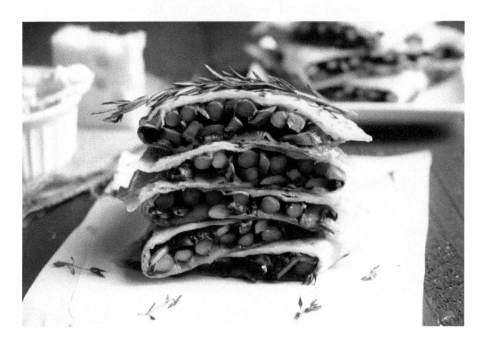

Prep Time: 15 minutes

Cooking Time: 15 minutes

Ingredients

- 4 English muffins

- 1/4 cup onion, finely minced

- 1 cup mushrooms, chopped

- 1 1/2 teaspoons oil

- 1/2 pound asparagus, trimmed and sliced crosswise into 1/2 inch rounds

- ½ teaspoon ground thyme or oregano or basil

- 1 ½ teaspoons vinegar

- Dash of salt and pepper

- ¾ cup mozzarella cheese, shredded (3 ounces)

Directions

- Toast muffin halves and place on a baking sheet in a single layer.

- In a large skillet over medium-high heat, sauté onions and mushrooms in oil, stirring often, until just beginning to brown.

- Add asparagus, seasoning, and vinegar. Sauté, stirring often, until asparagus is barely tender. Season lightly with salt and pepper.

- Divide the vegetable mixture equally onto the muffin halves. Top each muffin with shredded cheese.

- Broil muffins until the cheese melts. Watch carefully to avoid burning.

- Refrigerate leftovers within 2 hours.

Makes: 8 muffin halves

Nutritional Facts

Calories: 152 Sugar: 1.3 g Sodium: 742.8 mg Fat: 8.8 g Saturated Fat: 1.5 gUnsaturated Fat: 5.9 g Carbohydrates: 8.7 g Fiber: 3.1 g Protein: 10.7 g

2. <u>Autumn Squash Bisque With Ginger</u>

Prep Time: 15 minutes **Makes:** 10 cups

Cooking Time: 45 minutes

Ingredients

- 2 teaspoons oil

- 2 cups sliced onions

- 2 pounds winter squash, peeled, seeded, and cut into 2-inch cubes (4 generous cups)

- 2 pears, peeled, cored, and diced, or 1 can (15 ounces) sliced pears, drained and chopped

- 2 cloves garlic, peeled and crushed

- 2 Tablespoons coarsely chopped, peeled fresh ginger, or 1 teaspoon powdered ginger

- 1⁄2 teaspoon thyme

- 4 cups chicken or vegetable broth (see notes)

- 1 cup of water

- 1 Tablespoon lemon juice

- 1⁄2 cup plain nonfat yogurt

Directions

- Heat oil in a large pot over medium heat.

- Add onions and cook, stirring constantly until softened, 3 to 4 minutes.

- Add squash, pears, garlic, ginger, and thyme; cook, stirring, for 1 minute.

- Add broth and water; bring to a simmer.

- Reduce heat to low, cover, and simmer until squash is tender 35-45 minutes.

- Puree soup, in batches, if necessary, in a blender. (If using a blender, follow manufacturer's directions for pureeing hot liquids.)

- Return soup to pot and heat through. Stir in lemon juice.

- Garnish each serving with a spoonful of yogurt.

- Refrigerate leftovers within 2 hours.

Nutritional Facts

Calories: 80 Calories From Fat: 10 Total Fat: 1.5g Sodium: 340mg Carbohydrates: 18g Sugars: 6g Protein: 2g Dietary Fiber: 3g

3. **Baked Bean Medley**

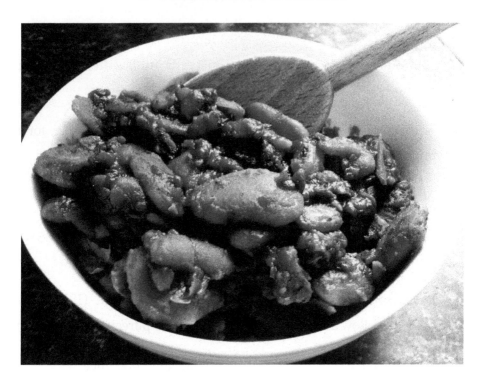

Prep Time: 15 minutes

Cooking Time: 1 1⁄2 hours

Makes: 8 cups

Ingredients

- 6 slices bacon

- 1 cup chopped onion

- 1 clove garlic, minced or 1/4 teaspoon garlic powder

- 1 can (15 ounces) pinto beans, drained and rinsed

- 1 can (15 ounces) great northern beans, drained and rinsed

- 1 can (16 ounces) kidney beans, drained and rinsed

- 1 can (15 ounces) garbanzo beans, drained and rinsed

- 1 can (15 ounces) pork and beans

- 3⁄4 cup ketchup

- 1⁄4 cup molasses

- 1⁄4 cup brown sugar

- 2 Tablespoons Worcestershire sauce

- 1 Tablespoon prepared mustard

- 1⁄4 teaspoon pepper

Directions

- Preheat oven to 375 degrees.

- Cut bacon into bite-sized pieces and place in skillet. Cook over medium heat (300 degrees in an electric skillet) until evenly browned. Remove from pan and set aside.

- Drain skillet, reserving 1 teaspoon of drippings. Add onion and garlic. Cook until onion is tender. Remove from skillet and add to bacon. Discard remaining drippings.

- Mix beans with bacon, onion, and garlic. Stir in remaining ingredients.

- Transfer to a 9x12 baking dish or 3-quart casserole dish. Bake in a preheated oven for 1 hour.

- Refrigerate leftovers within 2 hours.

- No bacon? Use 1 teaspoon cooking oil to saute vegetables.

Nutritional Facts

Calories 42 Calories from Fat 11.7 Total Fat 1.3g   Saturated fat 0.5g Sodium 32mg Carbohydrates 6.9g   Net carbs 6.5g Fiber 0.4g Glucose 3.3g Protein 0.5g

4. <u>Barley Summer Salad</u>

Prep Time: 10 minutes

Cooking Time: 45 minutes

Makes: 8 cups

Ingredients

- 1 cup dry barley

- 3 cups of water

- ¼ cup dried cranberries

- 1 cup fresh blueberries

- 1 cup sweet snap peas, chopped

- 2 cups apples or another fresh fruit or veggie, chopped (about 1 1/3 medium apples [3" diameter])

- ½ cup red bell pepper, seeded and chopped (about 1 small pepper)

- ½ cup green onions, sliced thin

- 1 Tablespoon vinegar

- 3 Tablespoons oil

- ¼ cup lemon or lime juice

Directions

- ❖ Place barley and water in a 2 or 3-quart saucepan. Bring to a boil, then turn to low. Cook covered for 45 minutes.

- ❖ Rinse cooked barley briefly in cold water. Drain.

- ❖ Add remaining ingredients. Toss well.

- ❖ Refrigerate leftovers within 2 hours.

Notes

- ❖ Substitute different fruits and vegetables in season.

- ❖ Add nuts or seeds for added protein.

Nutrition Facts

Calories 428 Calories from Fat 99 Fat 11g Saturated Fat 7g cholesterol 44mg Sodium 581mg Potassium 575mg Carbohydrates 68g Fiber 13g Sugar 6g Protein 16g Vitamin A 535IU

5. <u>Barley, Bean, And Corn Salad</u>

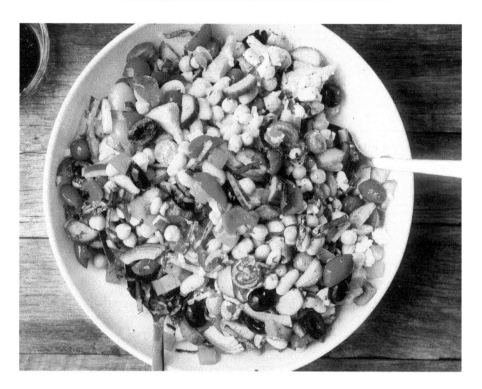

Prep Time: 15 minutes

Cooking Time: 45 minutes

Makes: 6 cups

Ingredients

- 2 cups cooked barley (cooking directions below)

- 1 can (15 ounces) kidney beans, drained

- 1 cup corn (canned and drained, frozen, or fresh cooked)

- 1 large red bell pepper, seeded and finely chopped

- ½ cup sliced celery

- ¼ cup sliced green onion

- 1 clove garlic, finely chopped or 1/4 teaspoon garlic powder

- ¼ cup fresh lemon or lime juice

- 2 tablespoons oil

- Salt and pepper to taste

- Fresh cilantro or parsley sprigs, for garnish (optional)

Directions

- Mix barley with remaining ingredients, except garnish, in a large bowl.

- Cover and chill several hours or overnight to allow flavors to blend.

- Garnish with cilantro or parsley sprigs, if desired, and serve.

- Refrigerate leftovers within 2 hours.

Nutrition Facts

Calories 256 Calories from Fat 72 Fat 8g Saturated Fat 1g holesterol 0mg Sodium 245mg Potassium 0 mg Carbohydrates 40g Fiber 9g Sugar 5g Protein 9g Net carbs 31g.

6. <u>Beef Barley Soup</u>

Prep Time: 15 minutes

Cooking Time: 45 minutes

Makes: 14 cups

Ingredients

- 1 pound lean ground beef (15% fat or less)

- 1 large carrot, diced, about 1 cup

- 1 small onion, diced, about 1 cup

- 2 stalk celery, diced, about 1 cup

- 2 cloves garlic, finely chopped or 1/2 teaspoon garlic powder

- 8 cups of water

- 2 teaspoons beef bouillon

- 1 can (14.5 ounces) diced tomatoes with juice

- 1 cup uncooked barley

- ½ teaspoon pepper

Directions

- In a large saucepot, cook ground beef over medium heat. Drain fat.

- Add carrots, onion, celery, and garlic; stir often and cook for about 5 minutes.

- Add 8 cups of water, bouillon, tomatoes with juice, barley, and pepper. Bring to a boil.

- Cover and reduce heat to a low boil. Cook for about 30 minutes or until barley is as tender as you like it.

- Serve immediately.

- Refrigerate leftovers within 2 hours.

Nutritional Facts

Calories 90 Calories from Fat 27 Total Fat 3g Cholesterol 11mg Sodium 728mg Carbohydrates 11g Net carbs 9.4g Fiber 1.6g Glucose .6g Protein 5g   Iron 0.2mg

7. **Bell Pepper Nachos**

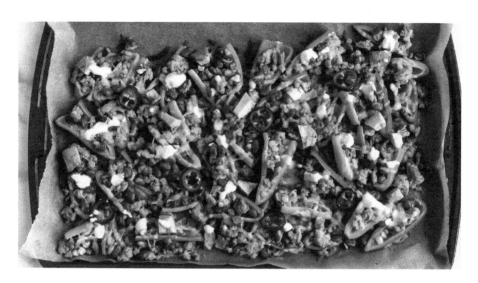

Prep Time: 5 minutes

Cooking Time: 15 minutes

Makes: 8 cups

Ingredients

- 4 bell peppers

- 1 cup of salsa

- 2 teaspoons seasoning (try a mixture-chili powder, garlic powder, ground cumin, pepper)

- 2 cups cooked meat (chopped or shredded), beans or tofu

- 1⁄2 cup shredded cheese

Directions

- Preheat oven to 350 degrees F.

- Wash bell peppers, remove seeds, and cut into bite-size pieces. Arrange pieces close together in a single layer on a large foil-lined baking sheet.

- In a medium bowl, combine salsa, seasonings and meat, beans, or tofu. Spoon the mixture evenly over pepper pieces then top with cheese.

- Bake for 15 minutes, or until peppers are heated through and cheese is melted. Serve warm.

- Refrigerate leftovers within 2 hours.

Nutrition Facts

Calories 764 Calories from Fat 405   Fat 45g

Saturated Fat 15g   Cholesterol 79mg   g

8. <u>Cherry Chicken Lettuce Wraps</u>

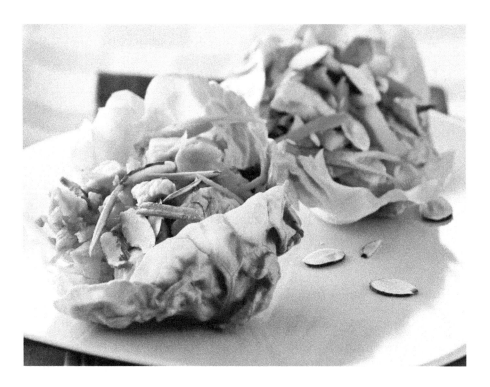

Preparation Time: 15 minutes

Cooking Time: 10 minutes

Servings: 1

Ingredients:

- 12 lettuce leaves
- 2 tbsp canola oil, separated
- ⅓ cup sliced almonds, toasted
- 1 ¼ lb chicken breast, the skin and bones removed and minced
- ½ cup green onion, diced

- 1 tbsp fresh ginger root, thinly cut
- 1 ½ cups carrots, roughly cut
- 2 tbsp rice vinegar
- 1 lb. dark sweet cherries, cut in halves and the pits removed
- 2 tbsp teriyaki sauce
- 1 tbsp honey

Directions:

- Set your stove to medium high heat and place a large sized skillet on it. Add 1 tbsp of oil to the pan and let it get hot. Put the skinless and boneless chicken in the pot and add your ginger. Sauté for 10 minutes. Be careful not to burn your chicken.
- You just want to make sure it is cooked through.
- Get a bowl and add honey, vinegar, 1 tbsp oil, and teriyaki sauce. Using a whisk, mix these ingredients well, before throwing in your almonds, the chicken mixture in your skillet, green onion, cherries and carrots.
- Using a spoon, place the mixture in the center of each of the twelve lettuce leaves.
- Roll the lettuce to cover this filling, and they are ready to serve.

Nutrition: Calories: 297 Carbohydrates: 21.5g Protein: 25g Fat: 12.4g

Sugar: 2g Sodium: 156mg Fiber: 1g

9. <u>Lamb, Butternut Squash and Date Tagine</u>

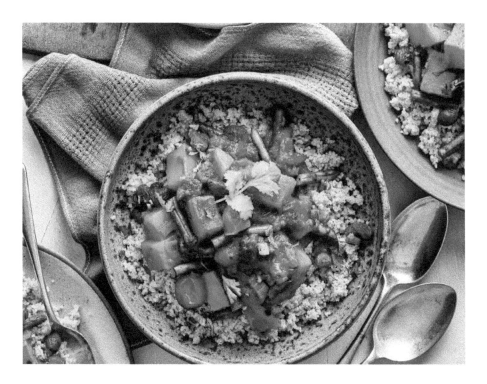

Preparation time: 5 minutes

Cooking time: 1 hour and 15 minutes

Servings: 4

Ingredients:

- 2 Tsps. coconut oil
- 1 Red onion, chopped
- 2cm ginger, grated
- 3 Garlic cloves, crushed or grated
- 1 teaspoon chili flakes (or to taste)
- 2 tsp. cumin seeds

- 2 teaspoons ground turmeric
- 1 cinnamon stick
- 800g lamb neck fillet, cut into 2cm chunks
- 1/2 tsp. salt
- 100g Medjool dates, pitted and sliced
- 400g Tin chopped berries, and half of a can of plain water
- 500g Butternut squash, chopped into 1cm cubes
- 400g Tin chickpeas, drained
- 2 tsp. fresh coriander (and extra for garnish)
- Buckwheat, Couscous, flatbread or rice to function

Directions:

- Pre heat the oven to 140C.
- Drizzle roughly 2 tbsps. coconut oil into a large ovenproof saucepan or castiron casserole dish.
- Add the chopped onion and cook on a gentle heat, with the lid for around five minutes, until the onions are softened but not too brown.
- Insert the grated ginger and garlic, chili, cumin, cinnamon, and garlic. Stir well and cook 1 minute with off the lid. Add a dash of water when it becomes too humid.
- Add from the lamb balls. Stir to coat the beef from the spices and onions, and then add the salt chopped meats and berries and roughly half of a can of plain water (100-200ml).
- Bring the tagine into the boil and put the lid and put on your skillet for about 1 hour and fifteen minutes.

- Add the chopped butternut squash and drained chickpeas. Stir everything together, place the lid back and go back to the oven to the last half an hour of cooking.
- When the tagine is able to remove from the oven and then stir fry throughout the chopped coriander.

Nutrition:

Calories: 317

Total Fat: 18 g

Total Carbohydrates: 14 g

10. <u>Avocado and Salmon Salad Buffet</u>

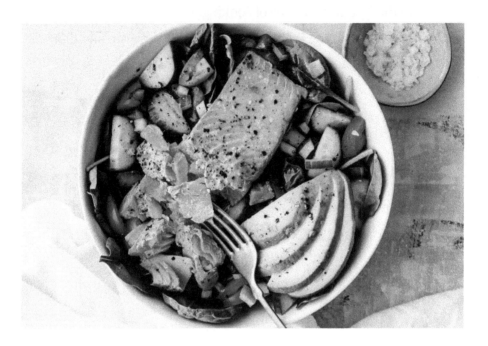

Preparation Time: 10 minutes

Cooking Time: 10 minutes

Servings: 2 - 3

Ingredients:

- ½ pieces cucumber
- 1 piece avocado
- ½ pieces red onion
- 250 g mixed salad
- 4 slices smoked salmon

Directions:

- Slice the cucumber and avocado into cubes and chop the onion. Spread the lettuce leaves on deep plates and spread the cucumber, avocado, and onion over the lettuce.
- Season with salt and pepper (you can also add a little olive oil to the salad).
- Place smoked salmon slices on top and serve.

Nutrition: Calories: 209 Cal Fat: 21 gCarbs: 33.19 g Protein: 8.82 g Fiber: 16.7 g

11. **Artichokes and Kale with Walnuts**

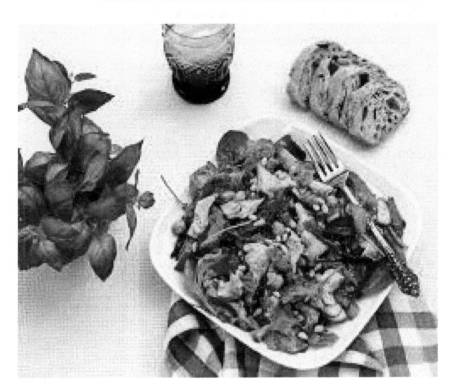

Total time: 40 minutes

Servings: 2

Ingredients:

- 1 cup of artichoke hearts
- 1 tbsp. parsley, chopped
- ½ cup of walnuts
- 1 cup of kale, torn
- 1 cup of Cheddar cheese, crumbled
- ½ tbsp. balsamic vinegar
- 1 tbsp. olive oil

- Salt and black pepper, to taste

Directions:

- Preheat the oven to 250°-270°F and roast the walnuts in the oven for 10 minutes until lightly browned and crispy and then set aside.
- Add artichoke hearts, kale, oil, salt, and pepper to a pot and cook for 20 to 25 minutes until done.
- Add cheese and balsamic vinegar and stir well. Divide the vegetables onto two plates and garnish with roasted walnuts and parsley.

Nutrition Facts: Calories: 152 kcal; Fat: 32g; Carbohydrates: 59g; Protein: 23g

12. <u>**Easy Korean Beef**</u>

Preparation Time: 10 minutes

Cooking Time: 10 minutes

Servings: 4

Ingredients:

- 1 tbsp sesame seeds
- 2 tsp sesame oil
- 2 tbsp green onion, diced
- 1 lb. lean ground beef
- 2 cups cauliflower rice
- 3 garlic cloves, thinly cut
- ¼ tsp ground black pepper
- ¼ cup soy sauce
- ¼ tsp ground ginger
- 1 tbsp coconut sugar

Directions:

- Make sure your stove is set to medium high heat and place a large skillet on it.
- Pour the sesame oil in the pan to make it hot, before adding garlic and ground beef.

- After 7 minutes, by which time the beef would crumble easily, turn down the stove to low and quickly continue with the following step.
- Grab a bowl and throw your black pepper, soy sauce, ginger, and coconut sugar in it. Using a whisk, mix these ingredients properly.
- Now, you can pour the coconut sugar mixture over the cooked beef that is still in the pan.
- Increase the heat back to medium and let the beef mixture simmer for about 3 minutes.
- Serve the keto Korean beef on top of your prepared cauliflower rice.
- Finally, garnish with sesame seeds and green onions.

Nutrition: Calories: 297 Carbohydrates: 8.9g Protein: 22.4g Fat: 13.3g

Sugar: 0.6g Sodium: 956mg Fiber: 3.7g

13. <u>Chicken with Sprouts Salad</u>

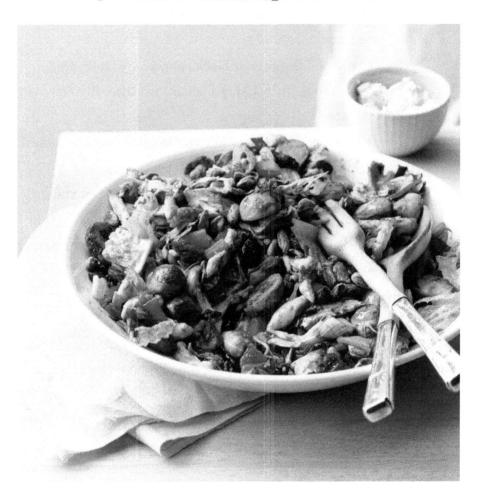

Total time: 50 Minutes

Servings:1

Ingredients:

- 8 oz. pork chops
- 1/8 tbsp. salt
- 1/2 tbsp. pepper,

- 1 tbsp. extra-virgin olive oil
- 1 tbsp. agave syrup
- 1 tbsp. Dijon mustard
- 6 oz. Brussels sprouts
- 1 garlic clove, crushed
- 1 handful parsley, chopped

Directions:

- Spray the chicken breast with cooking spray; sprinkle with salt and 1/4 tbsp. of the pepper. Whisk together oil, maple syrup, mustard, and 1/4 tbsp. pepper in a bowl.
- Add Brussels sprouts; toss to cover.
- Put the chicken breast on one side of a pan, and add Brussels sprouts on the other.
- Heat the oven (or air fryer) to 400°F and cook until the chicken is well colored and cooked through (15 to 18 minues).

Nutrition Facts: Calories 337 Fat 7g Protein 25g Carbohydrate 21g

14. __Ginger Asian Slaw__

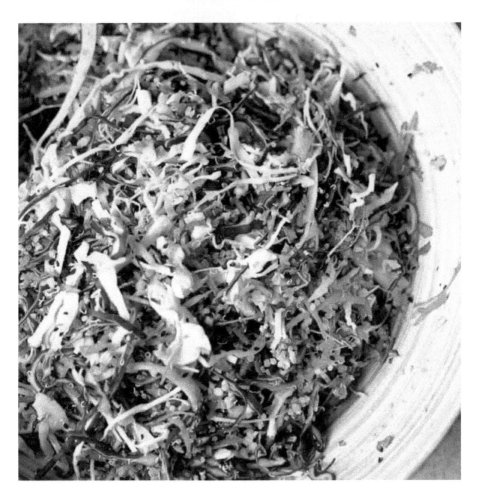

Preparation Time: 15 minutes

Cooking Time: 0 minutes

Servings: 8

Ingredients:

- Sea salt to your preferred taste
- 6 cups Napa cabbage, minced
- Pepper to your preferred taste
- 6 cups red cabbage, minced
- 3 tbsp lime juice
- 2 cups carrots grated
- 1 medium lime zest
- 1 cup cilantro, shredded
- ¼ tsp cayenne pepper
- ¾ cup diced green onions
- 1 garlic clove, thinly cut
- 1 tbsp extra virgin olive oil
- 1 ½ inch ginger, shredded
- 1 tbsp maple syrup
- 2 tbsp almond butter
- 1 tsp sesame oil
- 1 tbsp rice vinegar
- 1 tbsp apple cider vinegar
- 2 tbsp tamari

Directions:

- Into the cup of a blender add your olive oil, salt, pepper, maple syrup, lime juice, sesame oil, lime zest, apple cider vinegar, cayenne pepper, tamari, garlic rice vinegar, ginger, and almond butter.

- Blend these ingredients until you are left with a smooth mixture. This is your dressing.
- Next, you'll need a large mixing bowl. Put the cilantro, cabbage, green onions, and carrots inside it. Pour the mixture in your blender into the bowl and toss well.
- For about an hour, let the bowl stay in your fridge. The various flavors will meld deliciously and afterwards, you can serve.

Nutrition: Calories: 144 Carbohydrates: 12g

15. __Paleo-Force Bars__

Preparation Time: 15 minutes

Cooking Time: 10 minutes plus freezing time

Servings: 10

Ingredients:

- 10 pieces Medjoul dates (cored)
- 100 g Grated coconut
- 100 g crushed linseed
- 75 g Cashew nuts
- 60 g Coconut oil Directions:

Directions

- Put all ingredients in a food processor and pulse until a sticky and granular dough is formed. Line a small baking sheet with parchment paper.
- Spread the mixture on the bottom of the baking sheet and press down firmly.
- Let them solidify and harden them in the freezer for a few hours.
- After the mixture has hardened, cut it into bars.
- If you want to pack them as individual snacks, wrap the bars in cling film or baking paper.

Nutrition: Calories: 267 Cal Fat: 33.76 g Carbs: 89.14 g Protein: 18.2 g Fiber: 11.8 g

16.   <u>**Autumn Stuffed Enchiladas**</u>

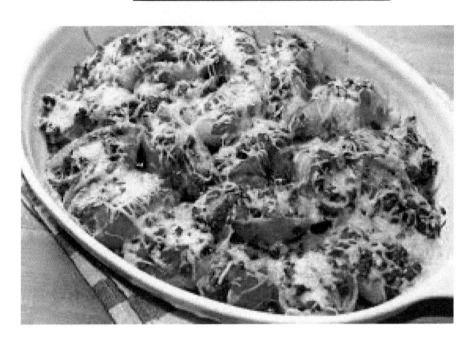

Total time:1 hour

Servings: 4

Ingredients:

- 1 lemon, juiced
- 1 cup cashews
- ½ oz. parsley
- 1 oz. roasted pumpkin seeds
- 8 corn tortillas
- 2 cups Butternut squash
- 1 cup salsa
- 1 can black beans
- 2 tbsp. olive oil

- ¼ tbsp. cayenne pepper
- 1 tsp. chili flakes
- 1 tsp. cumin
- 3 cloves garlic
- 1 jalapeno
- 1 red onion
- 1 cup Brussels sprouts

Directions:

- Soak the cashews in boiling water and set aside.
- Cut the squash in half, and after scooping out the seeds, lightly rub olive oil.
- Sprinkle with a little salt and pepper before putting on a baking sheet face down. Cook for about forty-five minutes at 400°F until it is cooked.
- Heat one tbsp. olive oil in a pan on medium heat and put chopped onion in, stirring until soft. Finely dice the jalapeno and garlic and finely slice the Brussel
- sprouts. Add these three things to the frypan and cook until the Brussels begin to wilt through.
- Strain and rinse the black beans, then add them to the frypan and mix well.
- When the squash is cooked and cool enough to handle, scrape out the soft insides away from the skin and put in a big bowl along with the Brussels mixture. Mix well again with salt and pepper to taste.
- Put the tortillas in the oven to soften up (don't let them get crispy)

- Spoon the squash mixture into the middle of the soft tortillas. Carefully roll them up to make little open-ended wraps, and then put in on a baking tray with the open ends down to stop them from unrolling.
- Do this for all twelve tortillas, then pour the rest of the salsa on top and spread to coat evenly.
- Change the temperature of the oven to 350°F and bake for 30 minutes.
- While these cooks put the drained, soaked cashews into a blender with one and a half cups cold water, lemon juice, and a quarter tsp. salt.
- Blend until smooth, adding water if it becomes too thick; this is your sour cream.
- When enchiladas are done, leave to cool while you chop parsley.
- Then drizzle the sour cream generously over the dish and top with parsley and pumpkin seeds.

Nutrition Facts: Calories: 333kcal; Fat: 11g Carbohydrate: 36g; Protein: 14g;

17. <u>Asian Chicken Drumsticks</u>

Total time: 36 Minutes Servings:2 Ingredients:

- 6 chicken drumsticks
- 1/4 cup rice vinegar
- 3 tbsp. agave syrup
- 2 tbsp. chicken stock
- 1 tbsp. lower-sodium soy sauce
- 1 tbsp. sesame oil
- 1 tbsp. tomato paste
- 1 garlic clove, crushed
- 2 tbsp. walnuts, chopped
- ½ tsp. turmeric

Directions:

- Put the chicken in a single layer in the oven and cook at 400°F until the skin is crispy (around 25to 28 minutes), turning drumsticks over partway through cooking.
- In the meantime, mix vinegar, stock, agave, soy sauce, oil, tomato paste, and garlic in a skillet. Bring to a boil over medium-high.
- Cook for about 6 minutes until thickened. Put the drumsticks and sauce in a bowl and toss to cover. Sprinkle with walnuts.

Nutrition Facts: Calories 488 Fat 30g Protein 25g Fiber 1g Sugars 26g

18.   <u>Zucchini Cream</u>

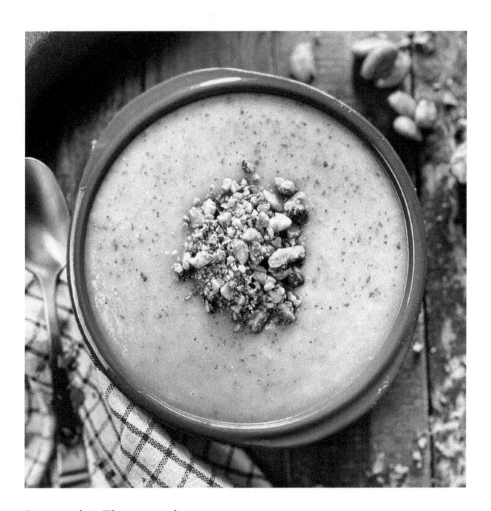

Preparation Time: 10 minutes

Cooking Time: 25 minutes

Servings: 8

Ingredients:

- 4 cups vegetable stock

- 2 tablespoons olive oil
- 2 sweet potatoes, peeled and cubed
- 8 zucchinis, chopped
- 2 onions, peeled and chopped
- 1 cup coconut milk
- A pinch of salt and black pepper
- 1 teaspoon dried rosemary
- 4 tablespoons fresh dill, chopped
- ½ teaspoon fresh basil, chopped

Directions:

- Heat a pot with the oil over medium heat, add the onion, stir, and cook for 2 minutes.
- Add the zucchinis and the rest of the ingredients except the milk and dill, stir and simmer for 20 minutes.
- Add the milk and dill, puree the soup using an immersion blender, stir, ladle into soup bowls and serve.

Nutrition: Calories: 324 Carbohydrates: 10g Protein: 14.8g Fat: 3g Sugar: 1.8g Sodium: 585mg Fiber: 0.4g

19. **<u>Vinaigrette</u>**

Preparation Time: 5 minutes

Cooking Time: 0 minutes

Servings: 1 cup

Ingredients:

- 4 teaspoons Mustard yellow
- 4 tablespoon White wine vinegar
- 1 teaspoon Honey
- 165 ml Olive oil

Directions:

- Whisk the mustard, vinegar, and honey in a bowl with a whisk until they are well mixed.
- Add the olive oil in small amounts while whisking with a whisk until the vinaigrette is thick.
- Season with salt and pepper.

Nutrition: Calories: 45 Cal Fat: 0.67 g Carbs: 7.18 g Protein: 0.79 g Fiber: 0.8 g

20. **Spicy Steak Rolls**

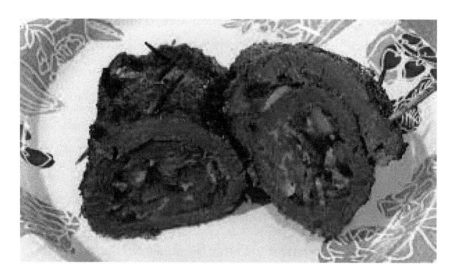

Preparation Time: 20 minutes

Cooking Time: 1 hour 15 minutes

Servings: 4

Ingredients:

- 10 slices bacon, chopped
- 1 (8 oz.) package fresh mushrooms, chopped
- 1 green bell pepper, chopped
- 1/2 small onion, chopped
- 1 clove garlic, minced, or to taste
- 4 beef round steaks
- 1/2 cup Montreal steak seasoning
- Toothpicks

Directions:

- In a large skillet, sauté bacon for about 10 minutes over medium-high heat until evenly browned.
- Add garlic, onion, green bell pepper, and mushrooms; sauté for about 10 minutes until mushrooms are tender. Put off the heat.
- Turn an outdoor grill to medium-high and lightly grease the grate.
- On a flat work surface, position a round steak between 2 pieces of plastic wrap.
- Use a meat tenderizer to flatten the steak. Do the same with the remaining steaks.

- Place Montreal steak seasoning into a shallow bowl. Dip 1 side of each steak into the seasoning and place on a cutting board, seasoning-side down.
- Spread some of the mushroom mixture over the center of each steak. Roll up and secure with toothpicks.
- Grill the rolled steaks for about 35 minutes on the preheated grill, turning once in a while, until they reach your desired doneness.
- Take off the toothpicks before serving.

Nutrition: Calories: 163 Carbohydrates: 45.6 g Protein: 3 g Fat: 0.6g

Sugar: 1g Sodium: 87mg Fiber: 0.7 g

21.   <u>Spicy Ras-El-Hanout Dressing</u>

Preparation Time: 10 minutes

Cooking Time: 5 minutes

Servings: 1 cup

Ingredients:

- 125 ml olive oil
- 1 piece lemon (the juice)
- 2 teaspoons honey
- 1 ½ teaspoon Ras el Hanout
- ½ pieces red pepper

Directions:

- Remove the seeds from the chili pepper.
- Chop the chili pepper as finely as possible.
- Place the pepper in a bowl with lemon juice, honey, and Ras-El-Hanout and whisk with a whisk.
- Then add the olive oil drop by drop while continuing to whisk.

Nutrition: Calories: 81 Cal Fat: 0.86 g Carbs: 20.02 g Protein: 1.32 g Fiber: 0.9 g

22.   Baked Potatoes With Spicy Chickpea Stew

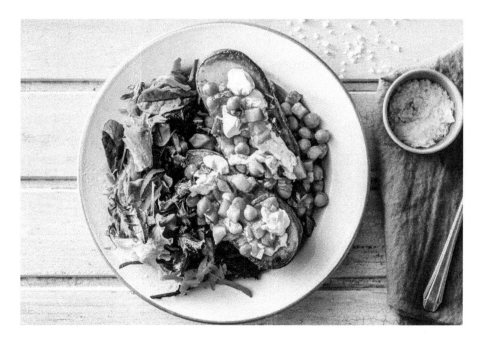

Total time: 70 minutes

Servings: 4

Ingredients:

- 4 baking potatoes, pricked around
- 2 tbsp. olive oil
- 2 red onions, finely chopped
- 4 tsp. garlic, crushed or grated
- 1-inch ginger, grated
- 1/2 tsp. chili flakes
- 2 tbsp. cumin seeds
- 2 tbsp. turmeric
- 2 tins chopped tomatoes

- 2 tbsp. cocoa powder, unsweetened
- 2 tins chickpeas – do not drain
- 2 yellow peppers, chopped

Directions:

- Preheat the oven to 400°F, and start preparing all ingredients. When the oven is ready, put in baking potatoes and cook for 50 minutes to 1 hour until they are done.
- While potatoes are cooking, put olive oil and sliced red onion into a wide saucepan and cook lightly, using the lid, for 5 minutes until the onions are tender but not brown.
- Remove the lid and add ginger, garlic, cumin, and cook for another minute on very low heat. Then add the turmeric and a tiny dab of water and cook for a few more minutes until it becomes thicker, and the consistency is ok.
- Then add tomatoes, cocoa powder, peppers, chickpeas with their water and salt. Bring to the boil, and then simmer on a very low heat for 45 to 50 minutes until it's thick.
- Finally, stir in the 2 tbsp. of parsley, some pepper and salt if you desire, and serve the stew with the potatoes.

Nutrition Facts: Calories: 520 Fat: 8g Carbohydrate: 91g Protein: 32g

23. Chicken Kofte with Zucchini

Total time: 52 Minutes

Servings:4

Ingredients:

- 1/2 cup low-fat Greek yogurt
- 2 tbsp. black olives, pitted and chopped
- 1 handful parsley, chopped
- 1/4 cup breadcrumbs
- 1/2 red onion, cubed
- 1 tbsp. ground cumin
- 1/8 tbsp. chili flakes
- 1-lb. ground chicken
- 4 tbsp. olive oil
- 4 zucchini, sliced

Directions:

- Mix yogurt, black olives, parsley, breadcrumbs, onion, 1/2 tbsp. salt, and 1/4 tbsp. pepper in a bowl, mixing with a whisk. Add chicken; blend in with hands.
- Shape chicken mixture into 8 patties. Heat 2 tbsp. olive oil in a skillet over medium heat. Add patties; cook 4 minutes on each side or until done.
- While kofte cooks, cook zucchini on a skillet. Brush them with 2 tbsp oil and season with the remaining pepper.

- Cook on high heat for 5 minutes, then season with salt. Serve 2 kofte per person with zucchini on the side.

Nutrition Facts: Calories 301 Fat 16.9g Protein 24g Carbohydrate 15g

24. Chipotle Citrus-Glazed Turkey Tenderloins

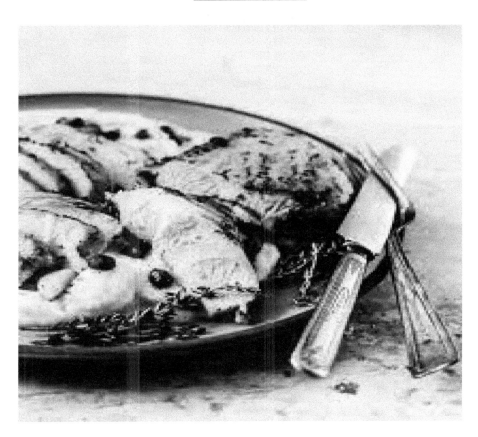

Total time: 25 Minutes

Servings:4

Ingredients:

- 4 5 oz. turkey breast tenderloins
- 1/4 tsp. salt
- 1/4 tsp. pepper
- 1 tbsp. extra-virgin olive oil

- 1 garlic clove, crushed
- 3/4 cup orange juice
- 1/4 cup lime juice
- 1 tsp. agave syrup
- 2 tsp. minced chipotle peppers
- 2 tbsp. parsley, chopped
- 1 bird's eye chili

Directions:

- Season turkey with salt and pepper. Cook it in a skillet with ½ tbsp. oil over high heat.
- Meanwhile, in a bowl, whisk the orange juice, lime juice, agave, ½ tbsp. oil, chipotle, and chili.
- Add the sauce to the skillet. Reduce heat and simmer for 14 to 16 minutes.
- Transfer turkey to a cutting board; let rest for 5 minutes. Simmer glaze until thickened, about 3 minutes. Slice the turkey, top with parsley, and serve with glaze.

Nutrition Facts: Calories 294 Fat 6g Protein 30g Carbohydrate 9g

25. **Coconut Shrimp**

Total time: 30 Minutes

Servings:2

Ingredients:

- 1/2 cup buckwheat flour
- 1 1/2 tbsp. pepper
- 2 eggs
- 2/3 cup coconut, shredded
- 1/3 cup panko (Japanese-style breadcrumbs)
- 12 oz. deveined shrimp, tail-on
- 1/4 cup agave syrup
- 1/4 cup lime juice
- 1 Bird's Eye chili, chopped
- 2 tbsp. parsley, chopped

Directions:

- Mix flour and pepper in a shallow dish. Gently beat eggs in another dish and mix coconut and panko in a third one.
- Holding each shrimp by the tail, dip them in flour, paing attention to not cover the tail; shake off excess.
- Dunk in egg, allowing any excess to trickle off. Dip in coconut blend and coat well.

- Put the shrimp in oven, and cook at 400°F until golden, 5 to 6 minutes, turning them over halfway through cooking. season with 1/4 tbsp. of the salt.
- While shrimp cook, whisk together nectar, lime juice, and serrano chile in a bowl.
- Sprinkle shrimp with parsley. Serve with sauce.

Nutrition Facts: Calories 250 Fat 9g Protein 15g Carbohydrate 30g

26. <u>Chicken with Broccoli & Mushrooms</u>

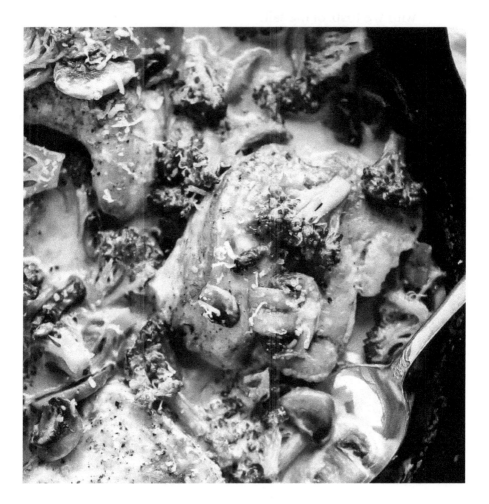

Preparation Time: 15 minutes

Cooking Time: 25 minutes

Servings: 6

Ingredients:

- 3 tablespoons olive oil
- 1-pound skinless, boneless chicken breast, cubed
- 1 medium onion, chopped
- 6 garlic cloves, minced
- 2 cups fresh mushrooms, sliced
- 16 ounces small broccoli florets
- ¼ cup water
- Salt and ground black pepper, to taste

Directions:

- Heat the oil in a large wok over medium heat and cook the chicken cubes for about 4–5 minutes.
- With a slotted spoon, transfer the chicken cubes onto a plate.
- In the same wok, add the onion and sauté for about 4–5 minutes.
- Add the mushrooms and cook for about 4–5 minutes.
- Stir in the cooked chicken, broccoli, and water, and cook (covered) for about 8–10 minutes, stirring occasionally.
- Stir in salt and black pepper and remove from heat.
- Serve hot.

Nutrition: Calories: 159 Carbohydrates: 40.3g Protein: 2g Fat: 2g

Sugar: 2.5g Sodium: 76mg Fiber: 0.3g

27. <u>Baked Root Veggies With Chili</u>

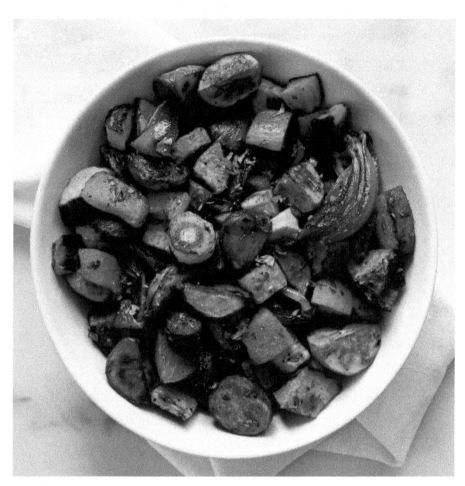

Total time: 70 minutes

Servings: 6

Ingredients:

- 3 Potatoes
- 3 Sweet potatoes
- 3 Yam

- 2 cups vegetable broth
- 1 can Red kidney beans
- 1 can white kidney beans
- 2 cans diced tomatoes
- 1 can black beans
- 1 tbsp. oregano
- 2 tbsp. paprika
- 1 tsp. cumin
- 2 tsp. chili powder
- 2 stalks celery
- 2 carrots
- 1 bell pepper
- 2 red onions
- 3 tbsp. Olive oil
- ½ oz. Parsley
- 2 avocados
- 1 bay leaf
- 1 can sweet corn
- 2 tomatoes
- 2 limes, juiced
- 1 head romaine

Directions:

- Scrub and fork the potatoes and yams. Drizzle them with oil. Sprinkle with salt and put on a baking tray for 45 minutes or until you can pierce easily with a knife.

- Heat the oil in a frying pan on medium heat and add the diced onion with the chopped bell pepper, diced carrots, celery, and a quarter tsp. of salt.
- Cook until the carrot is tender, then add the paprika, oregano, cumin, and chili powder.
- Put in tomato, the bay leaf, and the vegetable broth. Rinse the beans and drain well before adding to the pot.
- Stir well and leave to simmer for a further 30 minutes. After this time has passed, get a potato masher and mash the chili a few times to crush part of the beans and thicken the mixture.
- Add the juice of one lime and salt and pepper to taste.
- In a bowl, finely dice the avocado and lightly mash with salt, pepper, and the juice of another lime.
- In another bowl, drain and rinse the corn and toss in parsley, finely chopped, shredded romaine lettuce, a pinch of salt, and a tbsp. olive oil.
- Serve potatoes, chili, avocado, and salad so that everyone can assemble his/her masterpiece. Enjoy!

Nutrition Facts: Calories: 493kcal; Fat: 14g; Carbohydrates: 96g Protein: 14g;

28. <u>**Garlic Chicken Burgers**</u>

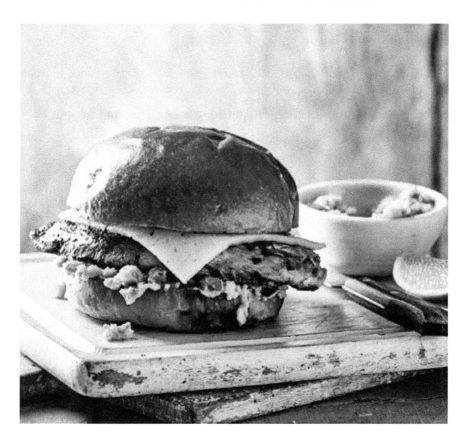

Total time: 30 minutes

Servings: 2

Ingredients:

- 10 oz. chicken mince
- ¼ red onion, finely chopped
- 1 garlic clove, crushed
- 1 handful of parsley, finely chopped
- 1 cup arugula

- ½ orange, chopped
- 1 cup cherry tomatoes
- 3 tsp. extra-virgin olive oil

Directions:

- Put chicken mince, onion, garlic, parsley, salt, and pepper to taste in a bowl and mix well. Form 2 patties and let rest 5 minutes.
- Heat a pan with olive oil, and when very hot, cook 3 minutes per side. Put the arugula on two plates; add cherry tomatoes and orange, dress with salt and the remaining olive oil.
- Put the patties on top and serve.
- These patties are delicious also when grilled. If you opt for grilling, just brush them with a bit of extra-virgin olive oil right before cooking.

Nutrition Facts: Calories: 353, Fat: 4.8g, Carbohydrate: 28.1g, Protein: 28.3g

29. **Shrimp with Kale**

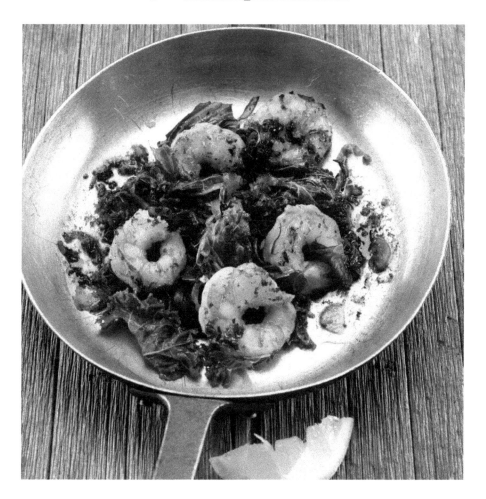

Preparation Time: 15 minutes

Cooking Time: 10 minutes

Servings: 4

Ingredients:

- 3 tablespoons olive oil
- 1-pound medium shrimp, peeled and deveined
- 1 medium onion, chopped
- 4 garlic cloves, chopped finely
- 1 fresh red chili, sliced
- 1-pound fresh kale, tough ribs removed and chopped
- ¼ cup low-sodium chicken broth

Directions:

- In a large non-stick wok, heat 1 tablespoon of the oil over medium-high heat and cook the shrimp for about 2 minutes per side.
- With a slotted spoon, transfer the shrimp onto a plate.
- In the same wok, heat the remaining 2 tablespoons of oil over medium heat and sauté the garlic and red chili for about 1 minute.
- Add the kale and broth and cook for about 4–5 minutes, stirring occasionally.
- Stir in the cooked shrimp and cook for about 1 minute.
- Serve hot.

Nutrition: Calories: 150 Carbohydrates: 34g Protein: 1g Fat: 0.3g Sugar: 1g Sodium: 93mg Fiber: 0g

30. <u>**Chicken Rolls With Pesto**</u>

Preparation Time: 15 minutes

Cooking Time: 20 minutes

Servings: 4

Ingredients:

- 2 tablespoon pine nuts
- 25 g yeast flakes
- 1 clove garlic (chopped)
- 15 g fresh basil
- 85 ml olive oil
- 2 pieces chicken breast

Directions:

- Preheat the oven to 175 ° C.
- Bake the pine nuts in a dry pan over medium heat for 3 minutes until golden brown.
- Place on a plate and set aside.
- Put the pine nuts, yeast flakes, and garlic in a food processor and grind them finely.
- Add the basil and oil and mix briefly until you get a pesto.
- Season with salt and pepper.
- Place each piece of the chicken breast between 2 pieces of cling film

- Beat with a saucepan or rolling pin until the chicken breast is about 0.6 cm thick.
- Remove the cling film and spread the pesto on the chicken.
- Roll up the chicken breasts and use cocktail skewers to hold them together.
- Season with salt and pepper.
- Melt the coconut oil in a saucepan and brown the chicken rolls over high heat on all sides.
- Put the chicken rolls in a baking dish, place in the oven and bake for 15-20 minutes until they are done.
- Slice the rolls diagonally and serve with the rest of the pesto.
- Goes well with a tomato salad.

Nutrition: Calories: 105 Cal Fat: 54.19 g Carbs: 6.53 g Protein: 127 g Fiber: 1.9 g

31.   <u>**Broccoli And Pasta**</u>

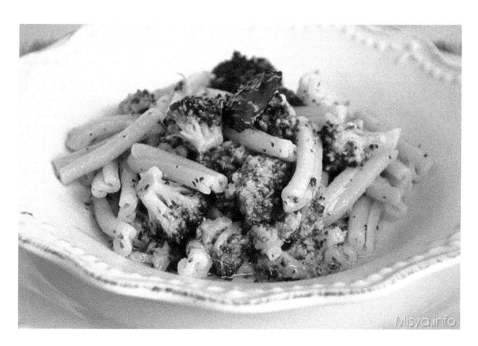

Total time: 30 minutes

Servings: 2

Ingredients:

- 5 oz. buckwheat spaghetti
- 5 oz. broccoli
- 1 garlic clove, finely chopped
- 3 tbsp. extra-virgin olive oil
- 2 scallions sliced
- ¼ tsp. crushed chilies
- 12 sage shredded leaves
- Grated Parmesan (optional)

Directions:

- Put broccoli in boiling water for 5 minutes, then add spaghetti and cook until both pasta and broccoli are done (around 8 to 10 minutes).
- In the meantime, heat the oil in a frying pan and add scallions and garlic.
- Cook for 5 minutes until it becomes golden.
- Mix chilies and sage to the pan and gently cook for 1 minute. Drain pasta and broccoli; mix with the scallion mixture in the pan. Add some Parmesan, if desired, and serve.

Nutrition Facts: Calories: 350 Fat: 8g Carbohydrate: 38g Protein: 6g

32. Buckwheat with Mushrooms and Green Onions

Total time: 50 minutes

Servings: 2

Ingredients:

- 1 cup buckwheat groats
- 2 cups vegetable or chicken broth
- 3 green onions, thinly sliced
- 1 cup mushrooms, sliced
- 2 tsp. extra-virgin olive oil

Directions:

- Combine all ingredients in a pot and cook on low heat for about 35 to 40min until the broth is completely absorbed.
- Divide between two plates and serve immediately.

Nutrition Facts: Calories 340kcal, Fat 10 g, Carbohydrate 51 g, Protein 11g

33. <u>**Herb and Cheese Burgers**</u>

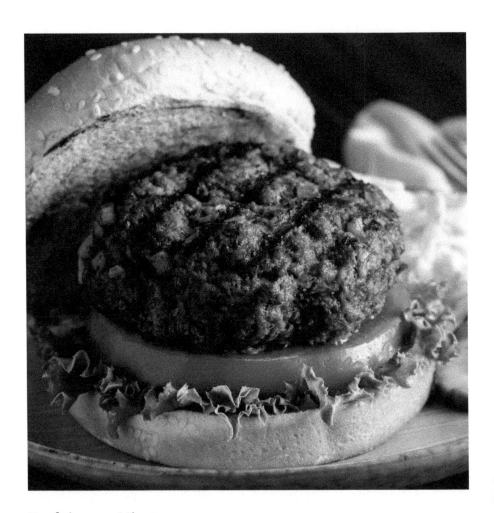

Total time: 25 Minutes

Servings: 4

Ingredients:

- 2 green onions, chopped
- ½ red onion, chopped

- 2 tbsp. parsley, chopped
- 4 tbsp. Dijon mustard
- 3 tbsp. breadcrumbs
- 1/2 tbsp. salt
- 1/2 tbsp. rosemary
- 1/4 tbsp. sage
- 1 lb. lean mincemeat
- 2 oz. cheddar, shredded
- 4 buckwheat burger buns

Directions:

- Preheat oven to 375°F. In a bowl, mix green onions, parsley, and 2 tbsp. mustard.
- In another bowl, mix breadcrumbs, red onion, sage, rosemary, and remaining 2 tbsp. mustard.
- Add mincemeat and mix well using a fork or the hands. Shape into 8 patties.
- Take one patty, put a tsp. of cheddar, and a tsp. of green onion blend.
- Top with another patty, and gently squeeze edges together to seal them well.
- Place burgers in a baking dish and cook 6 to 8 minutes. Serve burgers with buns, topped with arugula.

Nutrition Facts: 369 calories, 14g fat, 29g carbohydrate, 29g protein

34. **Kale Omelette**

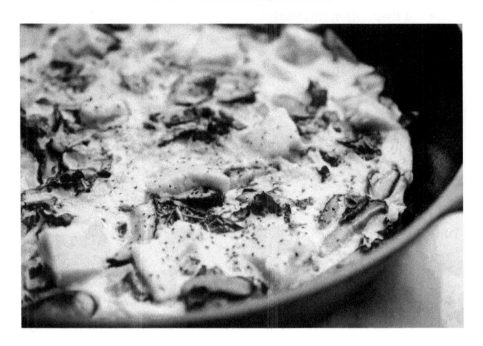

Total time: 15 minutes

Servings: 1

Ingredients:

- 2 eggs
- garlic clove
- handfuls kale
- 1 oz. goat cheese
- ¼ cup white onion, sliced
- teaspoons extra-virgin olive oil

Directions:

- Mince the garlic and finely shred the kale. Break the eggs into a bowl, add a pinch of salt. Beat until well combined. Place a pan over medium heat.
- Add 1 teaspoon of olive oil, add the onion and kale, cook for approx. 5 minutes, or until the onion has softened and the kale is wilted. Add the garlic and cook for another 2 minutes.
- Add 1 teaspoon of olive oil into the egg mixture, mix and add into the pan.
- Use your spatula to move the cooked egg toward the center and move the pan so that the uncooked egg mixture goes towards the edges.
- Add the cheese into the pan just before the egg is fully cooked, then leave for 1 minute.
- Serve immediately.

Nutrition Facts: Calories 219, Total Fat .6 g, Carbohydrate 7.7g,

Protein 8.2g

35. **Lemon-Fennel Spicy Cod**

Total time: 15 Minutes

Servings: 4

Ingredients:

- 3 tbsp. extra-virgin olive oil
- 2 garlic cloves, crushed
- 4 6-ounce cod fillets
- 2 cups fennel, finely sliced
- 1/4 cup red onion, chopped
- 2 tbsp. lemon juice
- 1 tbsp. parsley, chopped
- 1 tbsp. thyme leaves, chopped

Directions:

- Combine coriander, 2 tbsp. oil, garlic, salt, and pepper to taste in a bowl. Rub garlic blend over the cod fillets.
- Warm a skillet over medium-high heat.
- Add the cod and cook for 5 to 6 minutes on each side.
- In the meantime, add fennel, onion, lemon juice, 1 tbsp.oil, thyme, and parsley in a bowl, tossing to cover.
- Serve a plate of fennel salad with a cod fillet on top.

Nutrition Facts: Calories 259 Fat 9.7g Protein 36.3g Carbohydrate 5.3g

36. <u>Lime-Parsley Haddock</u>

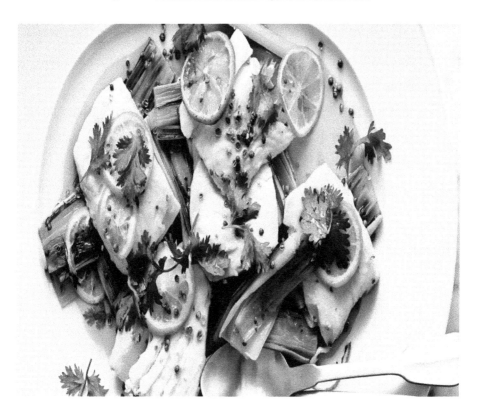

Total time: 50 Minutes

Servings:4

Ingredients:

- 4 6-oz. haddock fillets
- 1/2 tsp. salt
- 1/4 tsp. pepper
- 3 tbsp. extra-virgin olive oil
- 2 tbsp. parsley, chopped
- 1 tbsp. lime juice

- 1 tsp. lime zest

Directions:

- Preheat oven to 375°F. Mix the salt, pepper, 2 tsp. olive oil, lime juice, and zest in a bowl and whisk.
- Put the haddock fillets on a baking dish greased with cooking spray or one drop of extra virgin olive oil. Pour the sauce over the fish and cook 6 to 8 minutes until done.
- Top with parsley. Serve with a simple side of arugula seasoned with salt, pepper, and 1tbsp.olive oil.

Nutrition Facts: Calories 245 Fat 3g Protein 28g Carbohydrate 5g

37. **Rack of Lamb**

Preparation Time: 15 minutes

Cooking Time: 30 minutes

Servings: 2

Ingredients:

- 2 tbsps. All-purpose flour
- 1 tsp. salt
- 1/2 tsp. pepper
- 1 rack of lamb (1-1/2 lbs. an 8 ribs), trimmed
- 2 tbsps. Butter
- 1 cup white wine or chicken broth
- 1 tsp. grated lemon peel
- 1 garlic clove, minced
- 1/2 tsp. dried rosemary, crushed
- 1 bay leaf

Directions:

- In a shallow bowl, put pepper, salt and flour; coat lamb in flour mixture. Cook lamb in butter in a big skillet on medium high heat for 2 minutes per side; put onto a greased baking sheet.
- Bake without cover for 15-20 minutes at 375° till meat hits desired doneness (meat thermometer should read 170° for well-done, 160° for medium and 145° for mediumrare).

- Meanwhile, put bay lea, rosemary, garlic, lemon peel and wine in skillet; boil. Cook for 8 minutes till liquid reduces by half.
- Take away lamb from oven; loosely cover with foil. Stand before slicing for 5 minutes; serve lamb with sauce.

Nutrition: Calories: 644 Carbohydrates: 34g Protein: 1g Fat: 0.5g Sugar: 0.2g Sodium: 64mg Fiber: 0g

38. <u>Fried Chicken and Broccolini</u>

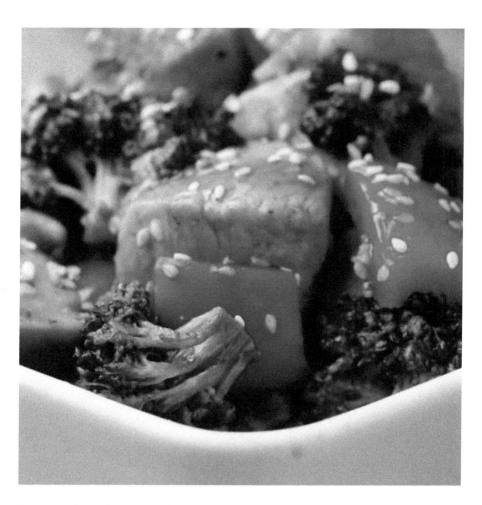

Preparation Time: 10 minutes

Cooking Time: 15 minutes

Servings: 5

Ingredients:

- 2 tablespoon coconut oil
- 400 g chicken breast
- Bacon cubes 150 g
- Broccolini 250 g

Directions:

- Cut the chicken into cubes.
- Melt the coconut oil in a pan over medium heat and brown the chicken
- with the bacon cubes and cook through.
- Season with chili flakes, salt, and pepper.
- Add broccolini and fry.
- Stack on a plate and enjoy!

Nutrition: Calories: 198 Cal Fat: 64.2 g Carbs: 0 g Protein: 83.4 g Fiber: 0 g

39. <u>Buckwheat with Onions</u>

Total time: 50 minutes Servings: 4

Ingredients:

- 3 cups of buckwheat, rinsed
- 4 red onions, chopped
- 1 white onion, chopped
- 5 oz. extra-virgin olive oil
- 3 cups of water
- Salt and pepper, to taste

Direction:

- Soak the buckwheat in warm water for around 10 minutes. Then add the buckwheat to your pot. Add in the water, salt, and pepper and stir well.
- Close the lid and cook for about 30-35 minutes until the buckwheat is ready.
- In the meantime, in a skillet, heat the extra-virgin olive oil and fry the chopped onions for 15 minutes until transparent and caramelized.
- Add some salt and pepper and mix well. Portion the buckwheat into four bowls or mugs. Then dollop each bowl with the onions. Remember that this dish should be served warm.

Nutrition Facts: Calories: 132; Fat: 32g; Carbohydrates: 64g; Protein: 22g

40. <u>Butternut Squash Alfredo</u>

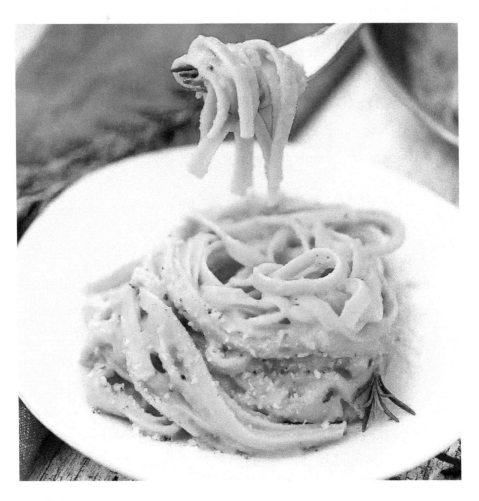

Total time: 40 minutes

Servings: 4

Ingredients:

- 9 oz. buckwheat linguine
- 2 cups vegetable broth

- 3 cups butternut squash, diced
- 1 tsp. paprika
- 2 cloves garlic
- 1 white onion
- 1 cup green peas
- 1 zucchini
- 2 tbsp. olive oil
- 2 tbsp. sage

Directions:

- Heat the oil in a frypan with medium heat. While it heats, ensures the sage leaves are clean and dry, then put in the oil to fry, moving around not to burn.
- Pull them out and put them on a paper towel.
- Into the frying pan, put the peeled and diced squash along with paprika, diced onion, and black pepper.
- Cook until the onion is soft, then add the broth and salt to taste.
- Bring to a boil before turning down to low heat and leaving the squash to cook through. In another pot, cook the linguine in water with a little salt.
- When the squash is tender, put it in a blender with all the liquid and other ingredients. Blend until creamy and taste to see if more salt, pepper, or spice is needed.
- Put it back in the frying pan to keep warm on low heat.
- Using a grater, grate the zucchini lengthwise to make long noodles. Make as many long ones as you can to blend in with the linguine.

- Add them to the sauce with the green peas and cook in the butternut squash for five minutes.
- When the pasta is done, save one cup of liquid before you drain it. Add the linguine to the pasta and stir well to coat the linguine.
- If the sauce is too thick, add a little pasta water. Serve the pasta topped with the fried sage leaves and a little blacker pepper.

Nutrition Facts: Calories: 432; Fat: 14g; Carbohydrate: 36g; Protein: 34g

41. **Caprese Skewers**

Total time: 15 minutes

Servings: 2

Ingredients:

- 4 oz. cucumber, cut into 8 pieces
- 8 cherry tomatoes
- 8 small balls of mozzarella or 4 oz. mozzarella cut into 8 pieces
- 1 tsp. of extra-virgin olive oil
- 8 basil leaves
- 2 tsp. of balsamic vinegar

Directions:

- Use 2 medium skewers per person or 4 small ones. Alternate the ingredients
- in the following order: tomato, mozzarella, basil, yellow pepper, cucumber, and repeat.
- Mix oil, vinegar, salt, and pepper and pour the dressing over the skewers.

Nutrition Facts:

Calories: 280 kcal, Fat: 8.6g, Carbohydrate: 14.4g, Protein: 17.2g

42. <u>Red Onion Frittata with Chili Grilled Zucchini</u>

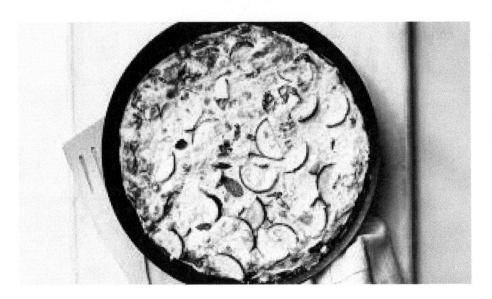

Total time: 35 minutes

Servings: 2

Ingredients:

- 1 ½ cups red onion, finely sliced
- 3 eggs
- 3 oz. cheddar cheese
- 2 tbsp. milk
- 2 zucchini
- 2 tbsp. oil
- 1 garlic clove, crushed
- ½ Bird's Eye chili, finely sliced
- 1 tsp. red wine vinegar

Salt and pepper to taste

Directions:

- Heat the oven to 350°F. Cut the zucchini into thin slices, grill them, and set them aside.
- Add 3 eggs, shredded cheddar cheese, milk, salt, and pepper.
- Whisk well and pour in a silicone baking tray and cook 25-30 minutes in the oven.
- Mix garlic, oil, salt, pepper, and vinegar and pour the dressing on the zucchini.
- Serve the frittata alongside the zucchini.

Nutrition Facts: Calories: 359, Fat: 7.8g, Carbohydrate: 18.1g, Protein: 21.3g

43. <u>Roasted Salmon with Fennel Salad</u>

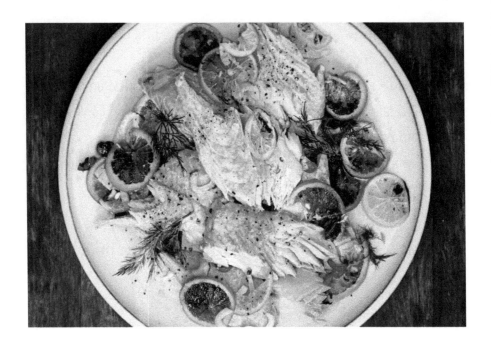

Total time: 25 Minutes

Servings:4

Ingredients:

- 2 tbsp. parsley
- 1 tbsp. thyme
- 4 6-oz. skinless salmon fillets
- 2 tbsp. extra-virgin olive oil
- 4 cups fennel, finely sliced
- 2/3 cup low-fat Greek yogurt
- 1 garlic clove, crushed
- 2 tbsp. orange juice

- 1 tbsp. lemon juice
- 2 tbsp. dill
- ½ tsp. turmeric

Directions:

- Preheat oven to 350°F. Mix parsley, thyme, salt, and pepper to taste in a bowl.
- Brush salmon with 1 tsp. oil; sprinkle the herb blend on top.
- Put salmon fillets on a baking dish, and cook at 350°F for 10 to 12 minutes until lightly brown on top.
- While salmon cooks, mix fennel, yogurt, garlic, dill, orange and lemon juice, salt,
- and pepper to taste in a bowl. Serve salmon fillets with the fennel salad on the side.

Nutrition Facts Calories 364 Fat 9g Protein 27g Carbohydrate 9g

44. <u>Casserole with Spinach and Eggplant</u>

Total time: 1 hour

Servings: 2

Ingredients:

- 1 eggplant
- 2 white onions
- 3 tbsp. extra-virgin olive oil
- 3 cups spinach, fresh
- 4 tomatoes
- 2 eggs
- ¼ cup almond milk, unsweetened
- 2 tsp. lemon juice
- 4 tbsp. parmesan

Directions:

- Preheat the oven to 400°F. Cut the eggplants, onions, and tomatoes into slices and sprinkle salt on the eggplant slices.
- Brush the eggplants and onions with olive oil and fry them in a grill pan.
- Cook spinach in a saucepan over moderate heat and drain in a sieve.
- Put the vegetables in layers in a greased baking dish: first the eggplant, then the spinach, and then the onion and the tomato.

- Repeat this. Whisk eggs with almond milk, lemon juice, salt, and pepper and pour over the vegetables.
- Sprinkle parmesan over the dish and bake in the oven for about 30 to 40 minutes.

Nutrition Facts: Calories: 446 kcal Fat: 31.82 g Carbohydrates: 30.5 g Protein: 13.95 g

45. <u>Salmon Fritters</u>

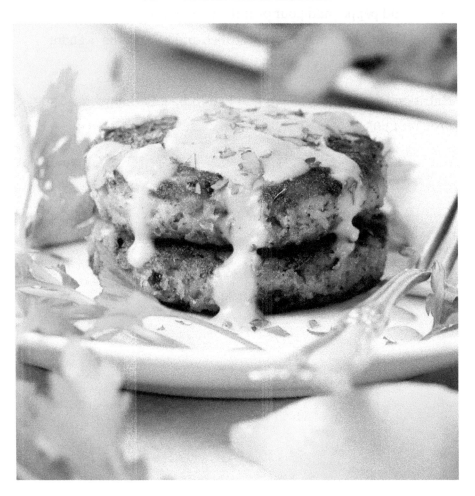

Total time: 30 minutes

Servings: 2

Ingredients:

- 6 oz. salmon, canned
- 1 tbsp. flour
- 1 garlic clove, crushed

- ½ red onion, finely chopped
- 2 eggs
- 2 tsp. olive oil
- Salt and pepper to taste
- 2 cups arugula

Directions:

- Separate egg whites from yolks and beat them until very stiff. In a separate bowl, mix salmon, flour, salt, pepper, onion, garlic, and yolks.
- Add egg whites and mix slowly. Heat a pan on medium-high. Add 1tsp. oil and, when hot, form salmon fritters with a spoon.
- Cook until brown (around 4 minutes per side) and serve with arugula salad seasoned with salt, pepper, and 1 tsp. olive oil.

Nutrition Facts: Calories: 320 Carbs: 18g Fat: 7g Protein: 27g

46. <u>**Spicy Chicken Breasts**</u>

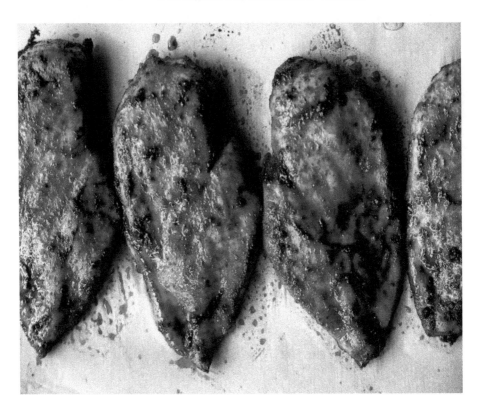

Total time: 25 minutes + 1 hour

Servings: 8

Ingredients:

- 2 cups buttermilk
- 2 tbsp. Dijon mustard
- 2 tbsp. hot pepper sauce
- 1-1/2 tbsp. garlic powder
- 8 chicken breast, skinless
- 2 cups buckwheat breadcrumbs

- 2 tbsp. extra-virgin olive oil
- 1/2 tbsp. paprika
- 1 pinch chili flakes
- 1/4 tbsp. oregano
- 1/4 tbsp. parsley
- 2 tsp. capers, finely chopped

Directions:

- Preheat Oven to 375°F. Marinate the chicken in buttermilk with mustard and hot sauce for at least 1 hour.
- Drain the chicken. Mix garlic, salt, paprika, chili flakes, oregano, parsley, and capers with breadcrumbs and coat the chicken.
- Put the chicken on a tray in a single layer. Cook for 18 to 20 minutes, turning one time halfway. Serve hot.

Nutrition Facts: 352 calories, 9g fat, 23g carbohydrate, 41g protein.

47. Chili Sweetcorn and Wild Garlic Fritters

Total time: 15 minutes

Servings: 4

Ingredients:

- ¾ cup rice flour
- 2 cups tinned or frozen sweetcorn
- 3 eggs
- 1 Bird's Eye chili, finely chopped
- Fry-light extra-virgin olive oil spray
- ¾ cup wild garlic leaves and bulbs, finely diced
- 2 cups lettuce, chopped

Direction:

- Mix the eggs, flour, chili, diced wild garlic, and sweetcorn in a bowl, season with the pepper and the salt.
- Spray a non-stick frypan and put it on medium heat.
- Use a spoon to scoop the egg mixture into the frypan batch by batch. The mixture will give you two large fritters per person or four small fritters.
- Fry the pancakes for about 4 minutes on one side, and then gently turn it to the other side and fry for another 3 minutes until it is set and golden brown.
- Serve immediately with salad.

Nutrition Facts: Calories: 198 Fat: 7g Carbohydrates: 30g Protein: 3g

Lightning Source UK Ltd.
Milton Keynes UK
UKHW050655090621
385195UK00004B/33